Create Your Great

AN INTERACTIVE JOURNAL

Luc Swensson

For information contact:
The Get It Factory Publishing House
2154 E Emerson Ave.
Salt Lake City, UT 84108

The Get It Factory
ryan@thegetitfactory.com

Please Visit:
www.ilovethislife.org
ISBN 978-1-953011-17-6

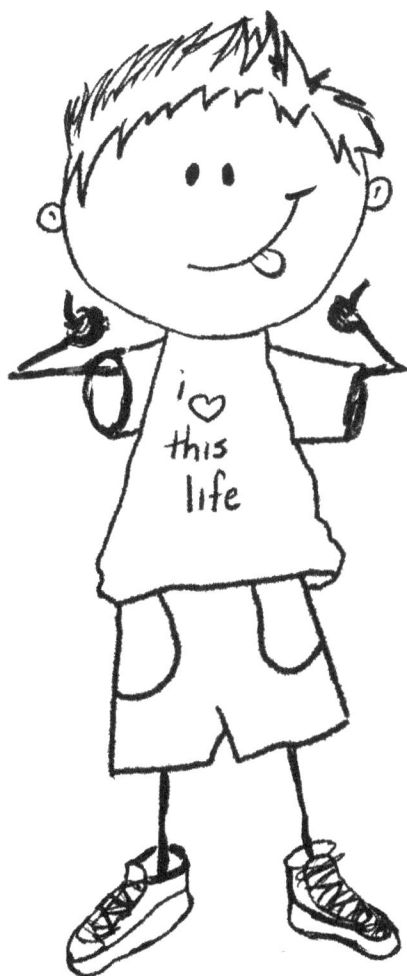

Thank You

I initially published this journal when I was just 13 years old. It was an accomplishment that exceeded my wildest expectations. To be honest, I never really imagined that I would be in a position to share my life's journey. But thanks to some incredible role models, I've been able to do just that.

Before we start our Create Your Great Journey, I'd like to say a few words about some of those incredible people.

Chris Lucas and Preston Brust of LoCash

None of this would be possible if it were not for you. Your music has changed my life. The power of your songs and the messages in your lyrics have not only given me the strength to believe in myself, but to create opportunities for others. I will forever be grateful for your support. Please keep writing and singing your songs, the world needs to hear them. I Love This Life! #musicmatters

Carly, Rick, Zizzly and Rich

I will never forget your kindness and support. You are responsible for the introduction to Chris and Preston and have been in my corner since the day I started my foundation. I owe you a lot, and I hope to someday return the favor. Your kind hearts and passion for others will always be a road map during my journey.

Brian Scott

You were my very first hero and role model. You taught me how to be my best both on and off the racetrack. I never missed a pre or post-race interview and no matter the situation you handled yourself in such a professional manner. You taught me that a platform in racing could lead to so many other opportunities to help people, and I strive every day to make you proud.

Tommy Mellott

You have become such an incredible role model for me. Your partnership with HOLO brand has allowed for so many kids to not only learn about mental health but be able to help others as well. You have inspired me to push even harder to help change the stigma around mental health. You have proven to me and so many others that dreams can come true.
GO CATS GO!!

My Dad

You are the one person that pushes me every single day to be my best. You have supported me in every crazy thing I have ever wanted to try and have encouraged me to never give up the fight. You have sacrificed everything for me and the pursuit of my dreams, and never once complained. You have lifted me up when I needed you most and you have always challenged me to be better.

I love you.

My Teachers

To all of my teachers over the years I can't thank you all enough. You have been such huge role models throughout all of my life and have put me on the right path and showed me anything is possible!

The Fighters

Your struggles, your stories and your perseverance to continue to fight is why I decided to start the I Love This Life Foundation. We all need inspiration, and we all need role models. For me, there is no better source than the Fighters. I promise to continue to fight right alongside you and do my part to see that everybody wins in the end.

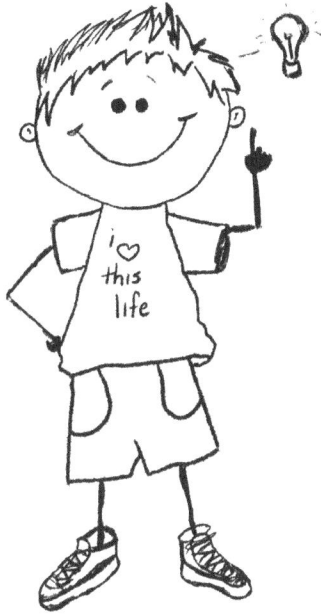

Ready?

Let's...

CREATE
YOUR
GREAT!

Hi! I'm Grafitti Luc.
Thanks for opening this journal!
I'm here to help you Create Your Great,
and this is the first step.

Tell me about your week.

i ♡ this life

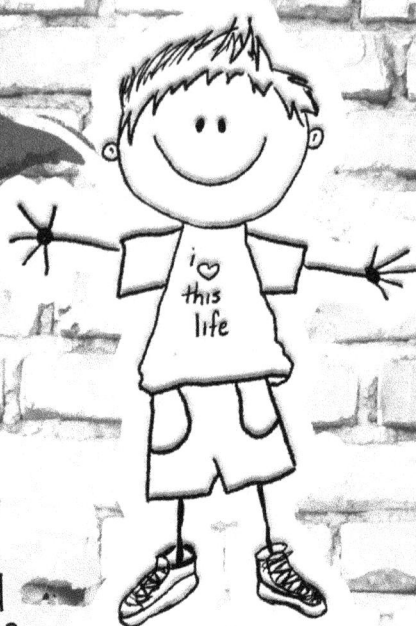

How did I make a difference this week?

Who inspired
me this week?
Why?

What is the best thing that happened
this week? How could this week
have been better?

Add your
own graffiti
here,

STOP OVERTHINKING.
YOU CAN'T CONTROL EVERYTHING.
JUST LET IT BE.

If you have someone joining you on your mission to Create Your Great, tell them to start here!

What is your name?
(Feel Free to add a small self portrait.)

How do you know your journal partner?

What happened this week to make you most proud of your journal partner?

What would you like to see your partner focus on next week?

EVERY DAY IS A NEW BEGINNING. TAKE A DEEP BREATH, SMILE, AND START AGAIN

Who inspired me this week? Why?

How did I make a difference this week?

What is the best thing that happened this week? How could this week have been better?

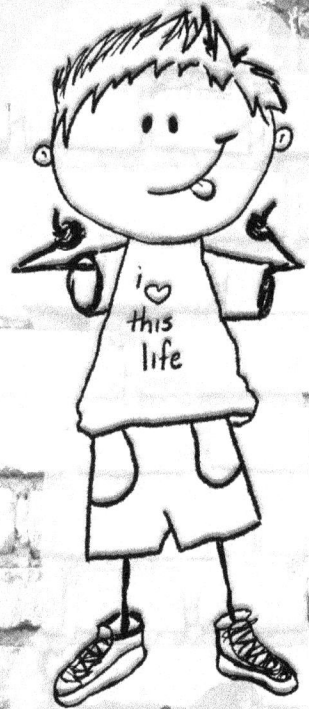

Add your own graffiti here,

Why was it a great week?

HEY!
You made it back for week 2.
You're definitely on your way
to creating your great!

What happened this week to make you most
proud of your journal partner?

How would
you describe
your journal
partner's
attitude
last week?

What would you like to see your partner focus on next week?

How did I make a
difference this week?

Who inspired
me this week?
Why?

What is the best thing that happened
this week? How could this week
have been better?

Add your own graffiti here,

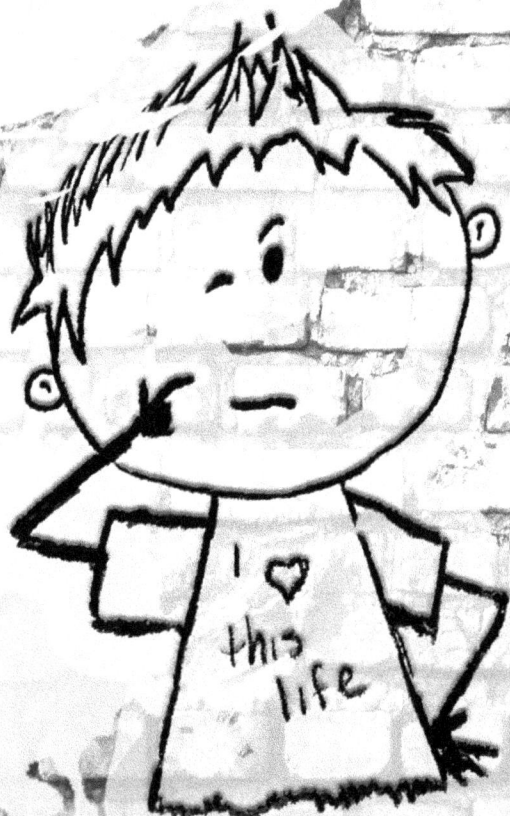

What happened this week to make you most proud of your journal partner?

How would
you describe
your journal
partner's
attitude
last week?

Why was it a great week?

I have a question
for you.

Do you know why Real Luc
decided to create these
journals?

What would you
like to see your partner
focus on next week?

ONE YEAR = 365 OPPORTUNITIES

Who inspired
me this week?
Why?

What is the best thing
that happened this week?

Add your own
graffiti here,

How did I make a difference this week?

Real Luc tells the
story all the time, so yo
may have already heard

I'll tell a quick versior
just in case.

What happened this week to make you most proud of your journal partner?

How would you describe your journal partner's attitude last week?

Why was it a great week?

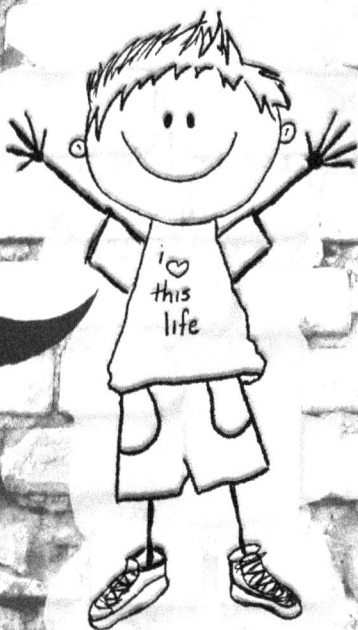

What would you like to see your partner focus on next week?

i ♥ this life

DON'T LOOK BACK,
YOU'RE NOT GOING THAT WAY.

How did I make a
difference this week?

Who inspired
me this week?
Why?

What is the best thing that happened
this week? How could this week have
been better?

Add your own graffiti here,

Real Luc was having a tough year.

School, family, and lots of other things just seemed like they were going wrong.

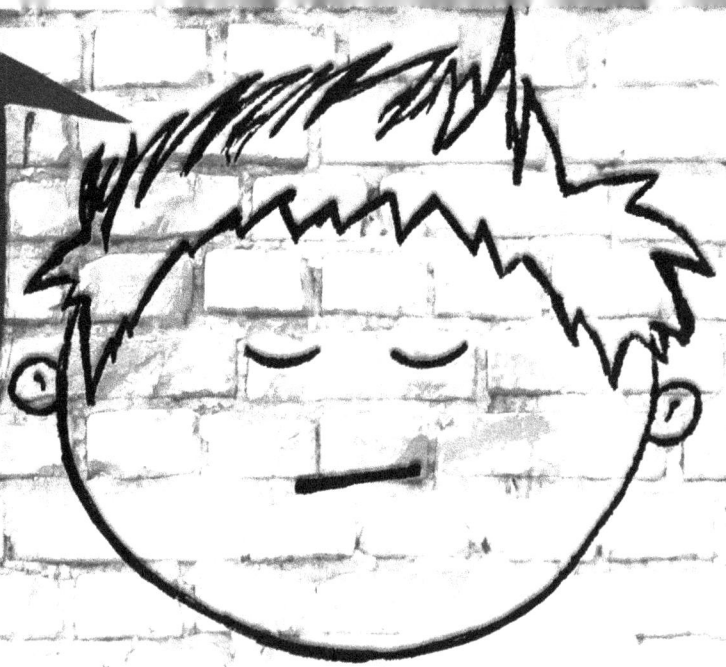

Why was it a great week?

How would you describe your journal partner's attitude last week?

What happened this week to make you most proud of your journal partner?

What would you like to see your partner focus on next week?

Add your own graffiti here,

How did I make a difference this week?

The worst point was when Real Luc decided to wear his new pink shoes to school.

What is the best thing that happened this week? How could this week have been better?

Who inspired me this week? Why?

What would you like to see
your partner focus on next week?

Why was it a great week?

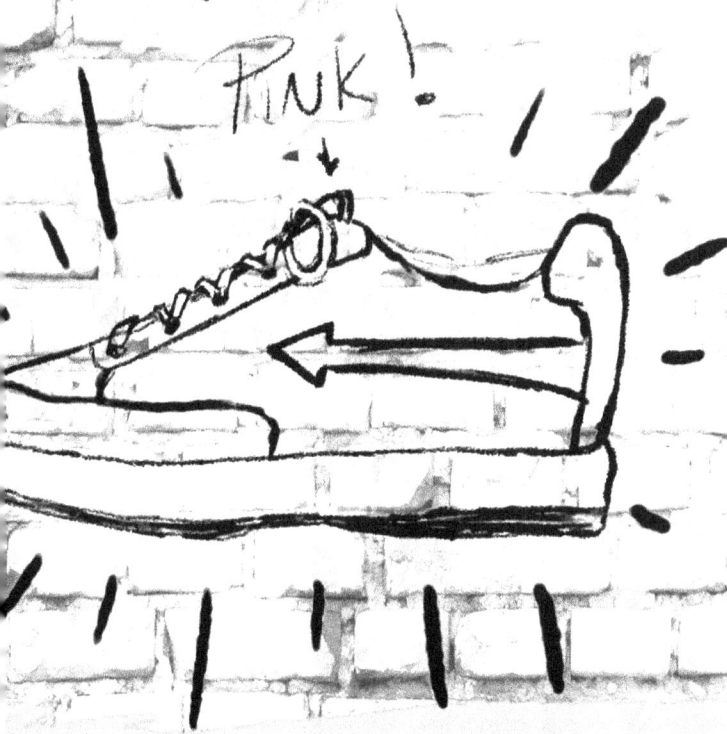

PINK!

How would you
describe your
journal partner's
attitude last week?

What happened this week to make you
most proud of your journal partner?

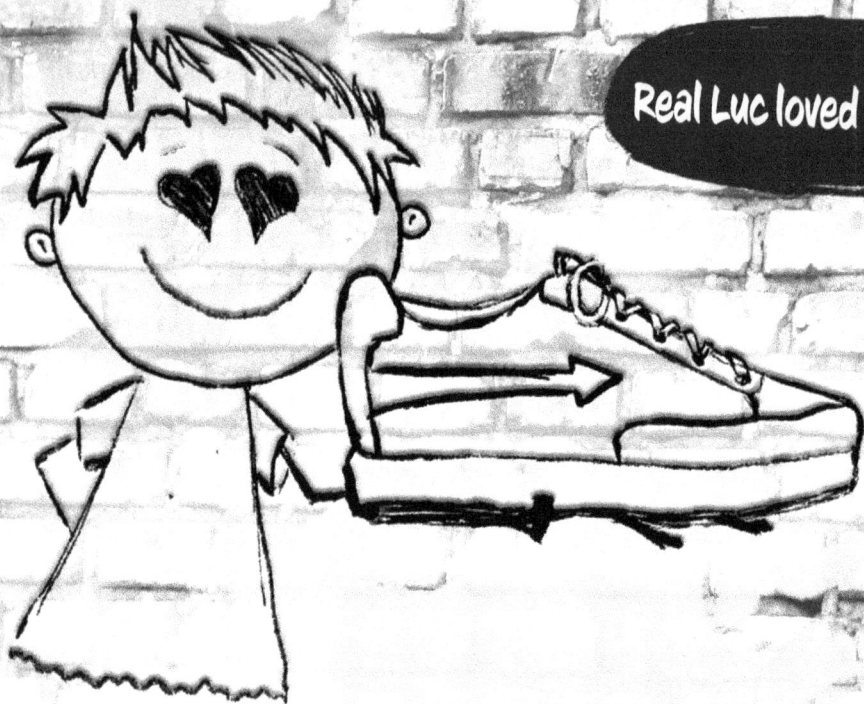

Let's switch it up a bit this week.
Instead of your normal graffiti, use this space to
design your perfect shoes.

What happened this week to make you
most proud of your journal partner?

How would you
describe your
journal partner's
attitude last week?

EVERY DAY MAY NOT BE GOOD...
BUT THERE IS SOMETHING
GOOD IN EVERY DAY

Why was it a great week?

What are your
all-time favorite
shoes?

What would you like to see
your partner focus on next week?

Even though Luc's shoes were super cool, when he wore them to school, kids bullied him almost nonstop.

Kids were making him feel bad about the shoes he loved.

How did I make a difference this week?

Add your own graffiti here,

What is the best thing that happened this week? How could this week have been better?

Who inspired me this week? Why?

How would you describe your journal partner's attitude last week?

Why was it a great week?

What would you like to see your partner focus on next week?

DON'T WORRY ABOUT FAILURES, WORRY ABOUT THE CHANCES YOU MISS WHEN YOU DON'T EVEN TRY.

What happened this week to make you most proud of your journal partner?

How did I make a difference this week?

Add your own graffiti here,

What is the best thing that happened
this week? How could this week
have been better?

Who inspired
me this week?
Why?

The bullying made an already difficult year even worse.

Why was it a great week?

How would you describe your journal partner's attitude last week?

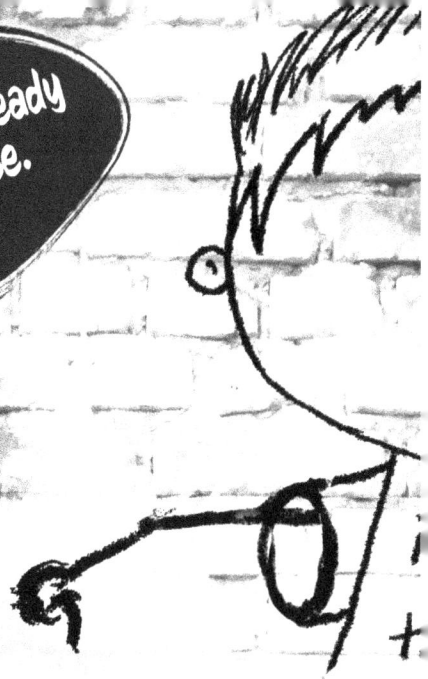

What happened this week to make you most proud of your journal partner?

NEVER GIVE UP ON YOUR DREAMS.

What would you like to see your partner focus on next week?

What is the best thing that happened this week? How could this week have been better?

Who inspired me this week Why?

Around the time when the bullying was at its worst, Real Luc's dad took him to a concert.

How did I make a difference this week?

Add your own graffiti here,

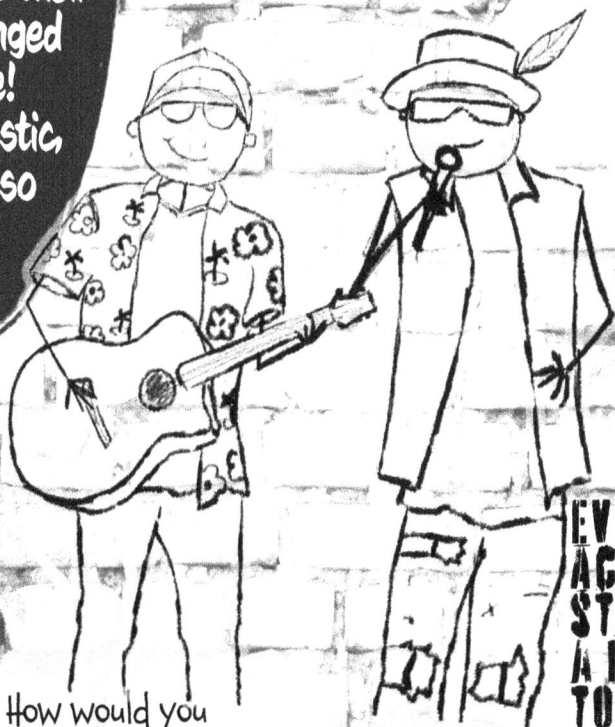

How did I make a
difference this week?

Add your own graffiti here

Who inspired me this week?
Why?

THE BEST WAY
TO PREDICT THE
FUTURE IS TO
CREATE IT.

What is the best thing that happened
this week? How could this week
have been better?

What would you like to see your partner focus on next week?

LoCash has a lot of great songs, but Luc especially loved one specific hit called, "I Love This Life."

What happened this week to make you most proud of your journal partner?

How would you describe your journal partner's attitude last week?

Why was it a great week?

How did I make a
difference this week?

Who inspired me
this week?
Why?

What is the best thing that
happened this week?
How could this week
have been better?

NEVER GIVE UP,
TODAY IS HARD,
TOMORROW MAY
BE WORSE,
BUT THE DAY AFTER THAT
WILL BE INCREDIBLE

Add your own graffiti here:

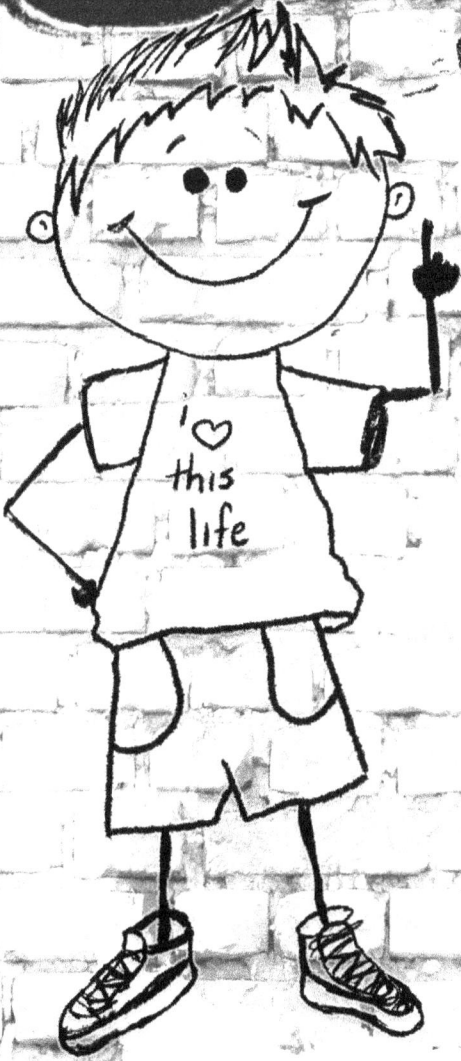

Shortly after the concert, Real Luc felt inspired.

What happened this week to make you most proud of your journal partner?

What would you like to see your partner focus on next week?

Why was it a great week?

How would you describe your journal partner's attitude last week?

Add your own graffiti here:

How did I make a difference this week?

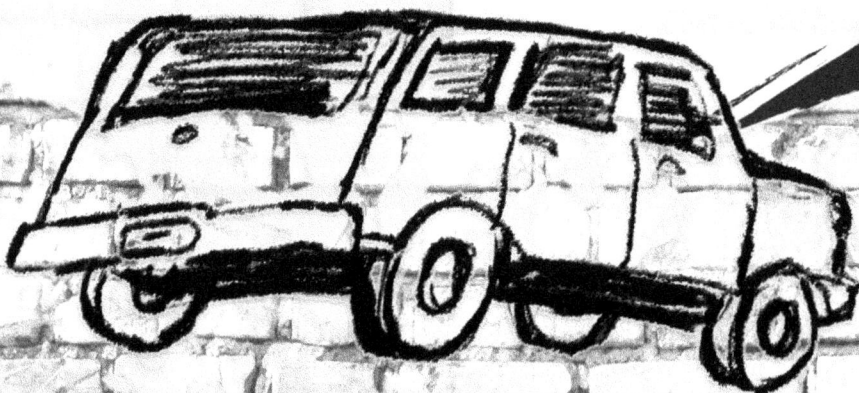

Who inspired me this week? Why?

What is the best thing that happened this week?

How could this week have been better?

On the way home, Luc shared his inspiration with his dad.

Why was it a great week?

Dad, I want to start an organization called "I Love This Life" to help kids who need help.

What would you like to see your partner focus on next week?

What happened this week to make you most proud of your journal partner?

DON'T SAY NEGATIVE THINGS IT GETS YOU NOWHERE.

How would you describe your journal partner's attitude last week?

How did I make a
difference this week?

Who inspired
me this week?
Why?

Add your own graffiti here:

ONE OF LIFE'S
GREATEST PLEASURES
IS DOING WHAT
PEOPLE SAY YOU
CANNOT DO.

What is the best thing
that happened this week?
How could this week have been better?

What happened this week to make you most proud of your journal partner?

Why was it a great week?

What would you like to see your partner focus on next week?

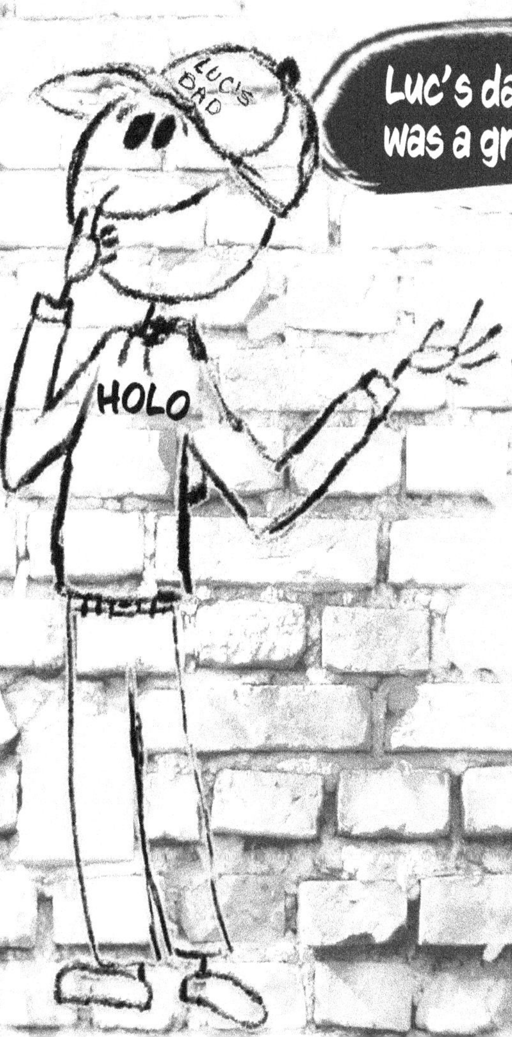

How would you describe your journal partner's attitude last week?

Add your own graffiti here:

How did I make a
difference this week?

They shared the idea
with the cool guys
from LoCash and
they also thought it
was a great idea!

Who inspired
me this week?
Why?

What is the best thing
that happened this week?
How could this week have been better?

THE FUTURE BELONGS TO
THOSE WHO BELIEVE
IN THE BEAUTY
OF THEIR DREAMS.

What would you like to see your
partner focus on next week?

What happened this week to make you most proud
of your journal partner?

How would you describe your
journal partner's attitude last week?

Why was it a great week?

If you could take a journey anywhere, where would you go?

Draw some of the things you might see on your dream journey.

At that moment, Real Luc started a journey that would chang his life, and the lives of many other kids.

Real Luc began telling his story to kids at schools and other events all over the courntry.

What would you like to see your
partner focus on next week?

How would you describe your
journal partner's attitude last week?

A SIMPLE HELLO
CAN LEAD TO MILLIONS
OF GOOD THINGS.

What happened this week to
make you most proud
of your journal partner?

Why was it a great week?

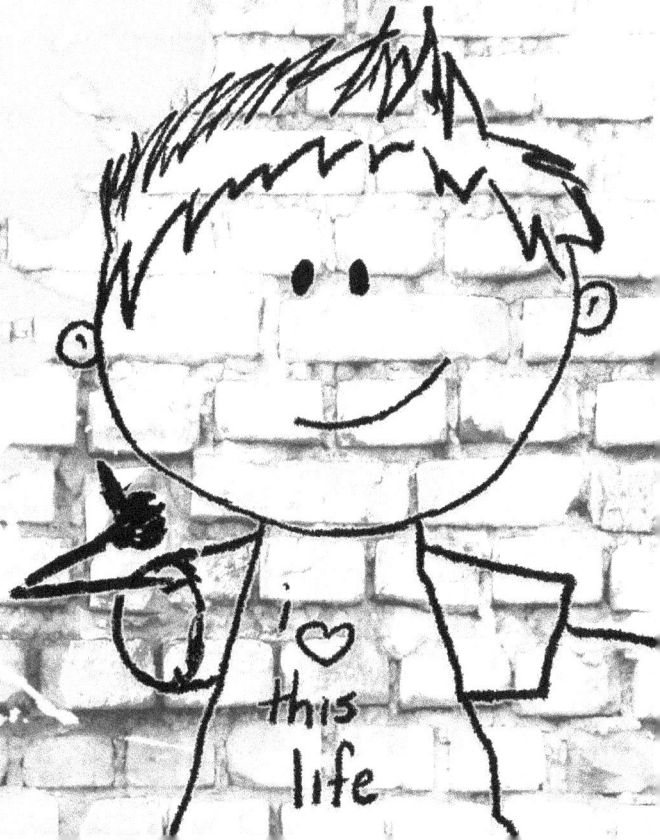

i ♡
this
life

Add your own graffiti here:

How did I make a difference this week?

What is the best thing
that happened this week?
How could this week have been better?

BIG THINGS OFTEN
HAVE SMALL BEGINNINGS

Who inspired
me this week?
Why?

What happened this week to make
you most proud of your journal partner?

Why was it a great week?

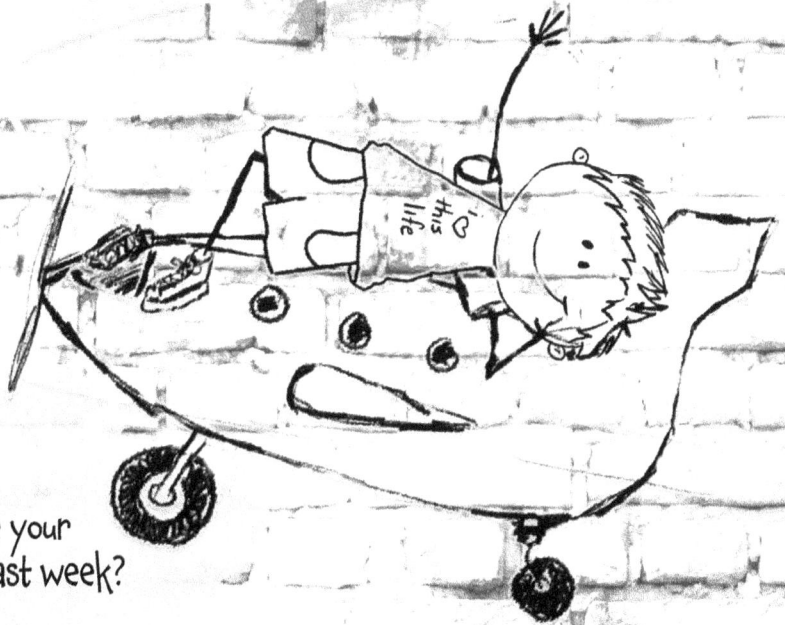

How would you describe your
journal partner's attitude last week?

What would you like to see your
partner focus on next week?

Luc and his dad met kids who were going
through many difficult, confusing, or just
wild times in thier lives.

Who inspired
me this week?
Why?

How did I make a difference this week?

Add your own graffiti here:

What is the best thing that
happened this week?
How could this week have
been better?

What happened this week to make
you most proud of your journal partner?

IF YOU CAN DREAM IT, YOU CAN DO IT...
NEVER GIVE UP.

In his travels, Real Luc found that kids seem
to feel better about things in their lives when
they learned they aren't alone. Luc shared
his story and other kids realized everyone in
the world is going through something, and
there will always be someone willing to help
them through anything.

Why was it a great week?

Real Luc has been introduced to some
amazing people and heard some
incredible stories.

What would you like to see your
partner focus on next week?

How would you describe your
journal partner's attitude last week?

This journal is a way to tell your story. Whether you share it or not, hopefully you can realize and help others by understanding none of us are alone.

Who can you go to if you need someone to talk to?
Draw the person, or something that reminds you of them here:

What do you like
most about talking to this person?

It works too! I'm going to share a couple of the stories Real Luc has heard on his travels. Maybe they'll help you, or someone you know.

How would you describe your journal partner's attitude last week?

What happened this week to make you most proud of your journal partner?

THE BEST PREPARATION FOR TOMORROW IS DOING YOUR BEST TODAY.

Why was it a great week?

What would you like to see your partner focus on next week?

How did I make a
difference this week?

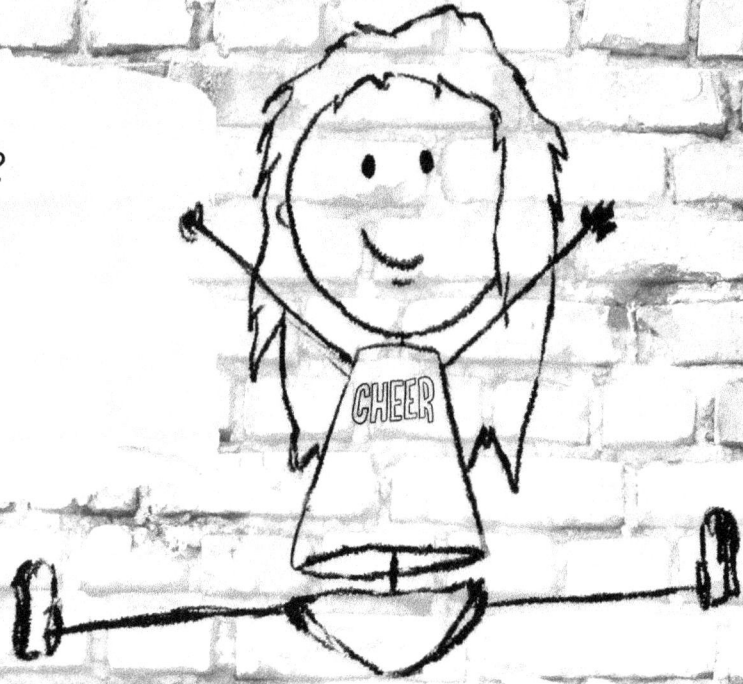

Who inspired
me this week?
Why?

What is the best thing that happened
this week? How could this week have
been better?

Add your own graffiti here,

This is my friend Perrey.

Well, its actually Graffiti Perrey, but she's based on Real Luc's real friend Perrey.

Why was it a great week?

DREAMS AND DEDICATION ARE A POWERFUL COMBINATION.

How would you describe your journal partner's attitude last week?

What happened this week to make you most proud of your journal partner?

What would you like to see your partner focus on next week?

How did I make a
difference this week?

When she was going into seventh
grade, Perrey's family decided
to move away from her home town.

They moved to a much bigger city.
It was very intimidating and scary.

Who inspired
me this week?
Why?

What is the best thing that happened
this week? How could this week have
been better?

Add your own graffiti here,

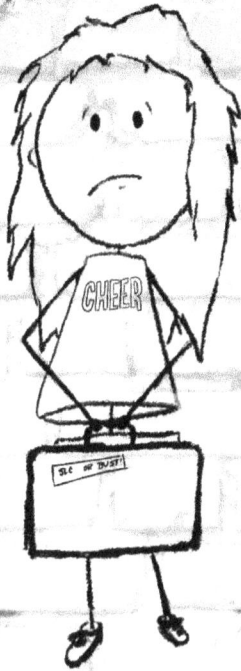

How would you describe your journal partner's attitude last week?

Why was it a great week?

START EACH DAY WITH A GRATEFUL HEART

What happened this week to make you most proud of your journal partner?

What would you like to see your partner focus on next week?

How did I make a
difference this week?

START EACH DAY
WITH A GRATEFUL
HEART

Who inspired
me this week?
Why?

What is the best thing that happened
this week? How could this week have
been better?

Add your own graffiti here,

What would you like to see
your partner focus on next week?

Why was it a great week?

Perrey had been an all-star
cheerleader for as long as
she could remember. She
was on her first cheer team
when she was just two years
old. Even with all of that
experience, she wasn't
confident she was good enough
to make a team in her new,
much bigger, city.

What happened this week to
make you most proud of your
journal partner?

How would you
describe your journal
partner's attitude
last week?

What is the best thing that happened this week? How could this week have been better?

Who inspired me this week? Why?

Add your own graffiti here,

She built up her courage and decided to go to tryouts.

Perrey did her best at the tryout...and she made the team

How did I make a difference this week?

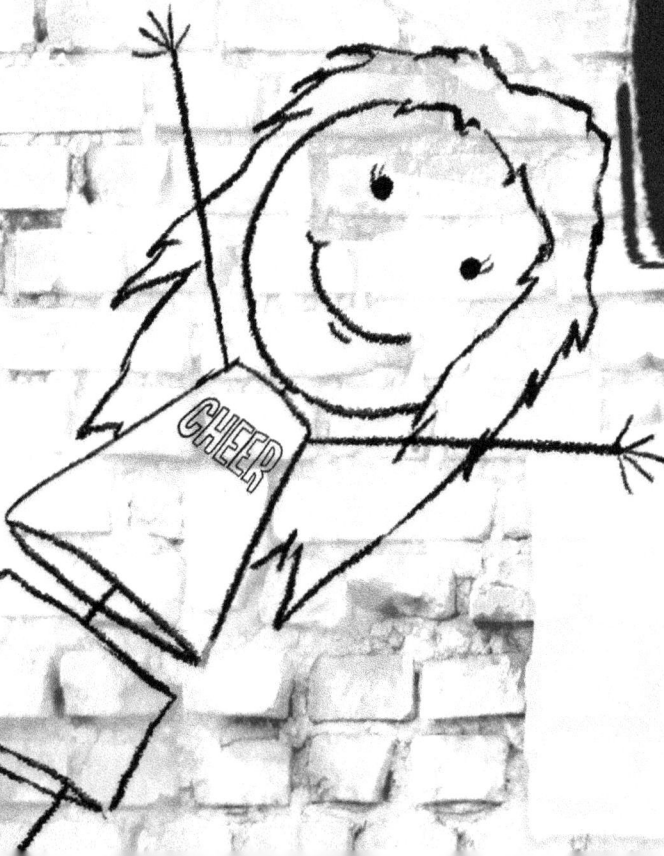

What happened this week to make you most proud of your journal partner?

What would you like to see your partner focus on next week?

HAPPINESS IS FOUND WHEN YOU STOP COMPARING YOURSELF TO OTHER PEOPLE

Why was it a great week?

How would you describe your journal partner's attitude last week?

LET YOUR SMILE CHANGE THE WORLD. DON'T LET THE WORLD CHANGE YOUR SMILE.

Who inspired me this week? Why?

What is the best thing that happened this week? How could this week have been better?

How did I make a difference this week?

Add your own graffiti here,

Unfortunately, making the team didn't make the move much easier.

Luckily, Perrey remembered listening to Luc and the messages he shared at her old school.

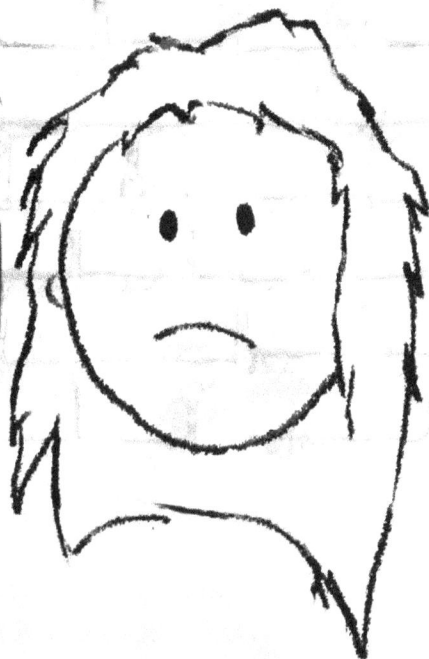

What happened this week to make you most proud of your journal partner?

Why was it a great week?

How would you describe your journal partner's attitude last week?

What would you like to see your partner focus on next week?

Have you had experiences with bullies?
If so, how did you handle the situation?

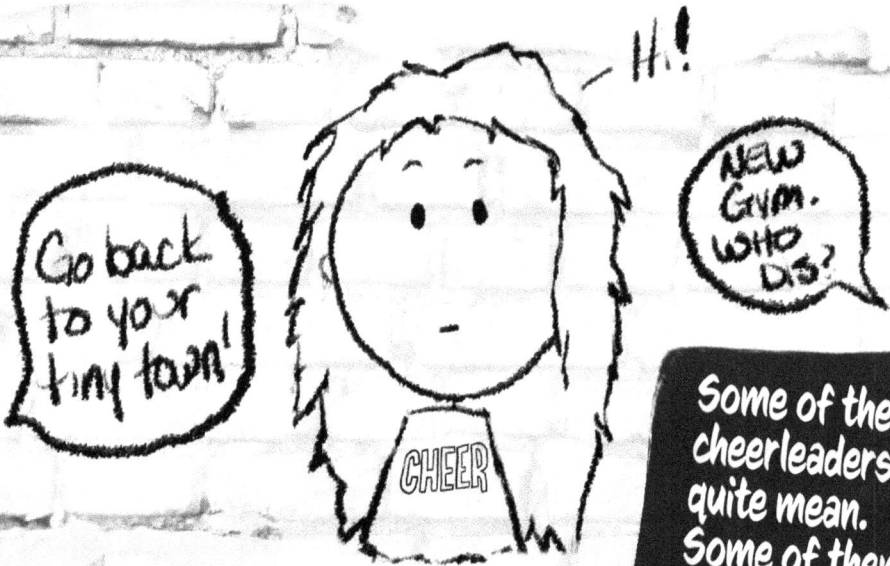

Draw a picture that shows
the emotions you felt:

How would you describe your journal partner's attitude last week?

Why was it a great week?

What happened this week to make you most proud of your journal partner?

DON'T COUNT THE DAYS, MAKE THE DAYS COUNT.

What would you like to see your partner focus on next week?

TRY TO BE A RAINBOW IN SOMEONE'S CLOUD.

How did I make a difference this week?

Who inspired me this week? Why?

What is the best thing that happened this week? How could this week have been better?

Add your own graffiti here,

Perrey didn't let the bullies stop her. She worked as hard as she could.

Still, something just didn't feel quite right.

Why was it a great week?

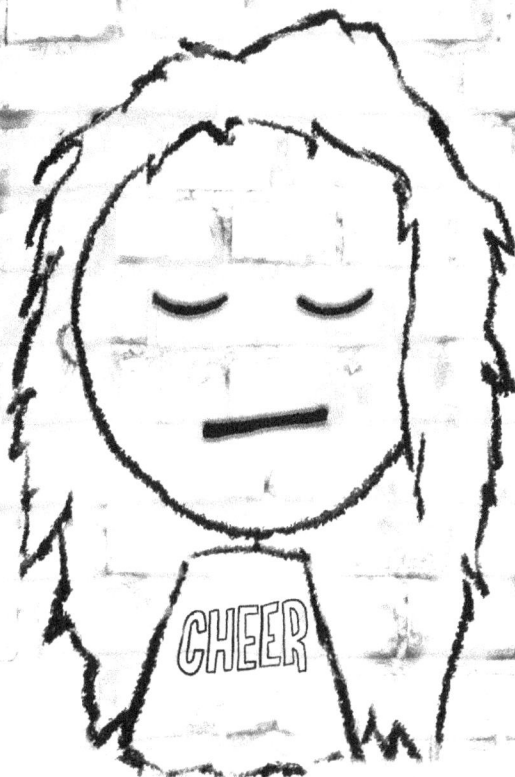

CHEER

How would you describe your journal partner's attitude last week?

What happened this week to make you most proud of your journal partner?

What would you like to see your partner focus on next week?

Who inspired me
this week? Why?

Even though she never missed
a practice and worked until she
was exhausted, she wasn't getting
better at the tumbling and cheer
stunts. In fact, she felt like she
was getting worse somehow.

She also felt tired all the time,
and just never really felt like hersel

How did I make a
difference this week?

What is the best thing that happened
this week? How could this week have
been better?

Add your own graffiti here,

Why was it a great week?

WHEN YOU FEEL LIKE QUITTING, THINK ABOUT WHY YOU STARTED.

How would you describe your journal partner's attitude last week?

What happened this week to make you most proud of your journal partner?

What would you like to see your partner focus on next week?

Add your own graffiti here,

Who inspired me this week? Why?

What is the best thing that happened this week? How could this week have been better?

How did I make a difference this week?

Finally, her parents decided to take her to the doctor to try to find out why Perrey was feeling so off.

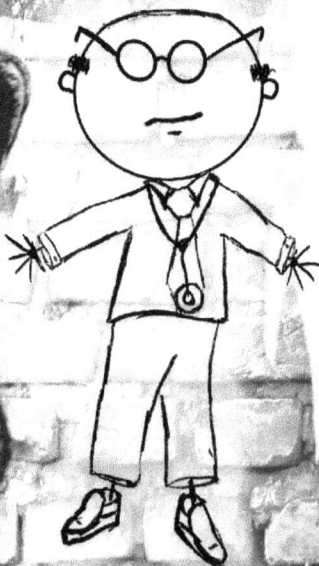

How would you describe your journal
partner's attitude last week?

What happened this week to make you
most proud of your journal partner?

BE THE CHANGE YOU
WISH FOR IN THE WORLD.

What would you like to see
your partner focus on next week?

Why was it a great week?

Add your own graffiti here,

What is the best thing that happened this week? How could this week have been better?

Who inspired me this week? Why?

**YOU ONLY FAIL.
IF YOU STOP TRYING.**

How did I make a difference this week?

How would you describe your journal partner's attitude last week?

What happened this week to make you most proud of your journal partner?

What would you like to see your partner focus on next week?

Why was it a great week?

The doctor sent Perrey directly to the hospital. where doctors and nurses were waiting for her.

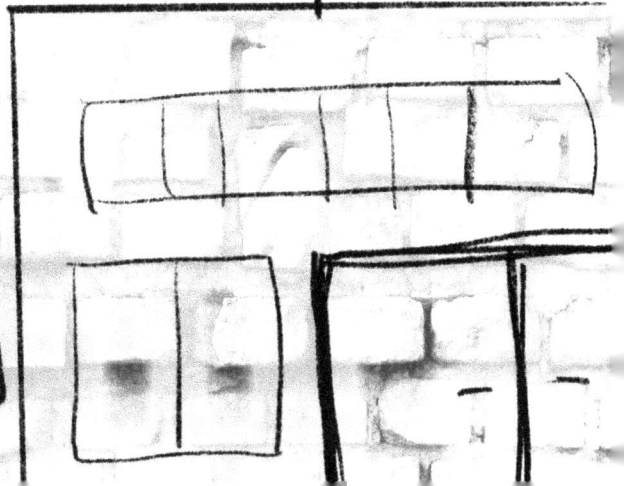

CHILDR

HOSPI

EMERGENCY

What is the best thing that happened this week? How could this week have been better?

Add your own graffiti here,

Who inspired me this week? Why?

How did I make a difference this week?

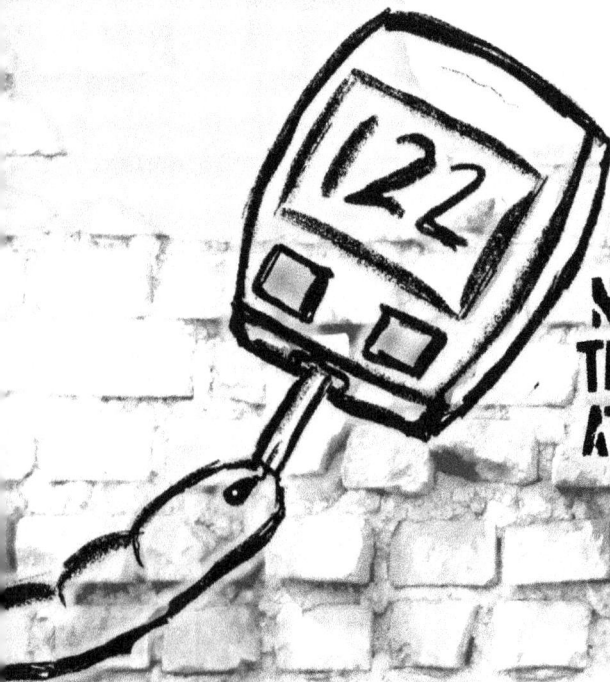

NO ONE EVER HURT THEIR EYES LOOKING AT THE BRIGHT SIDE.

How would you describe your journal partner's attitude last week?

What would you like to see your partner focus on next week?

Why was it a great week?

Perrey was diagnosed with Type 1 Diabetes and was very sick. She had to spend the next few days in the hospital to get her blood sugar regulated and learn to take care of herself now that she knew she had a lifelong disease.

What happened this week to make you most proud of your journal partner?

Perrey learned how to track her blood sugar and give herself shots of medicine to keep her from getting sick again.

Draw a picture or a comic strip that shows a challenge you have to overcome in your life:

What happened this week to make you most proud of your journal partner?

How would you describe your journal partner's attitude last week?

What would you like to see your partner focus on next week?

Why was it a great week?

BE THE REASON SOMEONE SMILES TODAY

Who inspired
me this week?
Why?

What is the best thing
that happened this week?

Add your own
graffiti here,

How did I make a difference this week?

Perrey's parents
were worried about
her because
of everything she
was going through.

hat happened this week to make you
nost proud of your journal partner?

How would
you describe
your journal
partner's
attitude
last week?

Why was it a great week?

What would you
like to see your partner
focus on next week?

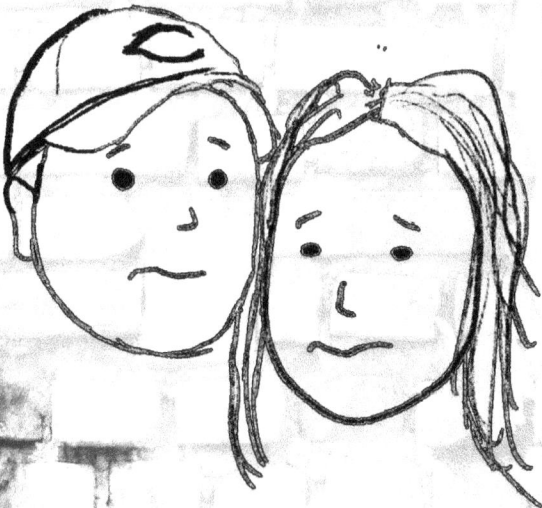

What is the best thing that happened this week?

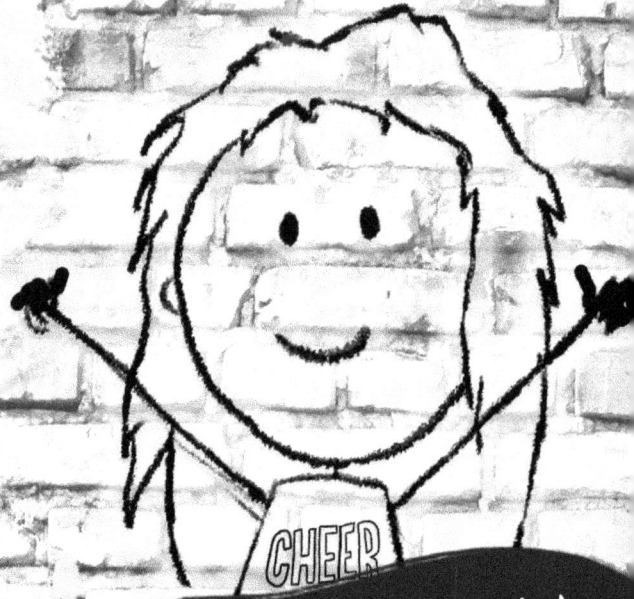

How did I make a difference this week?

Add your own graffiti here,

Perrey wasn't worried at all.

Remember, she heard Luc speak before, and she knew there are always people out there to help her as long as she keeps working hard.

CHEER

Who inspired me this week? Why?

How would you describe your journal partner's attitude last week?

What would you like to see your partner focus on next week?

Why was it a great week?

What happened this week to make you most proud of your journal partner?

ALWAYS REMIND YOURSELF TO FOCUS ON HAPPINESS, SUCCESS AND MOTIVATION.

How did I make a difference this week?

What is the best thing that happened this week?

Add your own graffiti here,

Two days after getting out of the hospital, Perrey took her new bag of needles, medication, and apple juice to the cheer gym and she practiced like nothing had ever happened.

Who inspired me this week? Why?

What would you
like to see your partner
focus on next week?

Why was it a great week?

LIGHT TOMORROW
WITH TODAY.

What happened this week to make you
most proud of your journal partner?

How would you
describe your journal
partner's attitude
last week?

Who are some of the people
who help you LOVE THIS LIFE?

BE THE SUNSHINE
WHEN SKIES ARE GREY.

Draw some of your favorite things.
Things that make you LOVE THIS LIFE!

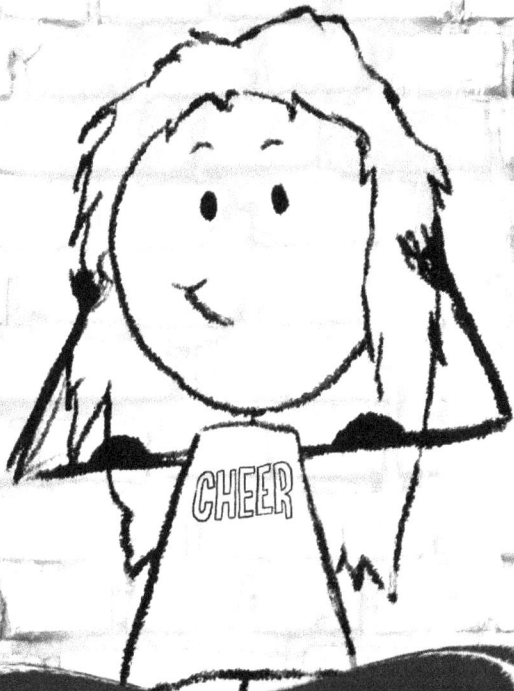

What would you like to see your partner focus on next week?

Perrey wasn't going to let diabetes hold her back because...SHE LOVES THIS LIFE!!

What happened this week to make you most proud of your journal partner?

How would you describe your journal partner's attitude last week?

Why was it a great week?

What is the best thing that happened this week? How could this week have been better?

Who inspired me this week Why?

Real Luc has another friend who always loved sports, but mostly, he always loved fooball!

How did I make a difference this week?

Add your own graffiti here,

What would you like to see
your partner focus on next week?

Why was it a
great week?

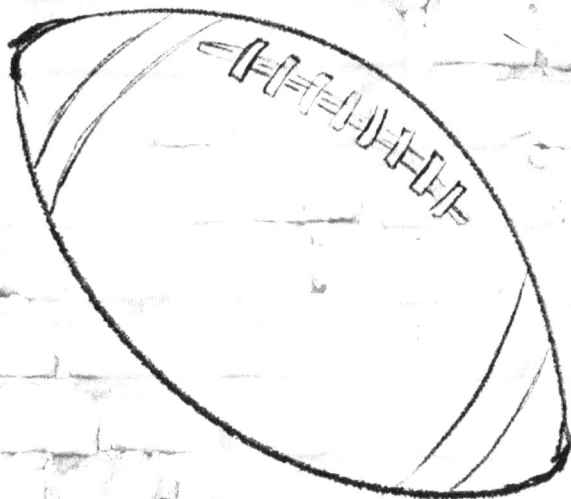

How would you
describe your
journal partner's
attitude last week?

STAY STRONG.
STAND UP.
HAVE A VOICE.

What happened this week
to make you most proud
of your journal partner?

What do you want to be when you grow up?

This friend wanted to be a quarterback.

Draw a picture of how you think you'll look when you go to work:

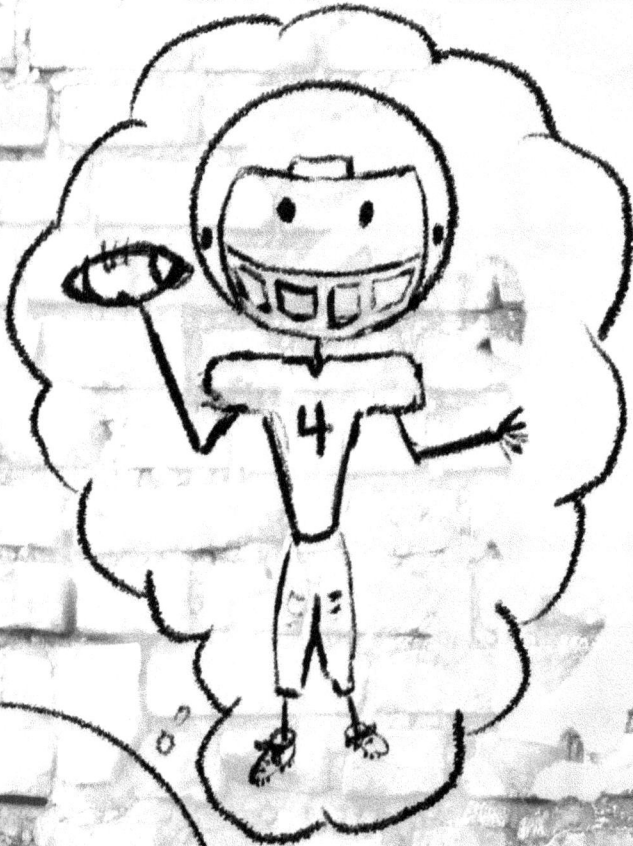

Why was it a
great week?

What would you like to see
your partner focus on next week?

**BELIEVE
IN
YOURSELF!**

How would you
describe your
journal partner's
attitude last week?

What happened this week to make you
most proud of your journal partner?

Add your own graffiti here:

How did I make a
difference this week?

What is the best thing
that happened this week?
How could this week have been better?

Who inspired
me this week?
Why?

What would you like to see your partner focus on next week?

In fact, he wanted to be a Division 1 college football starting quarterback.

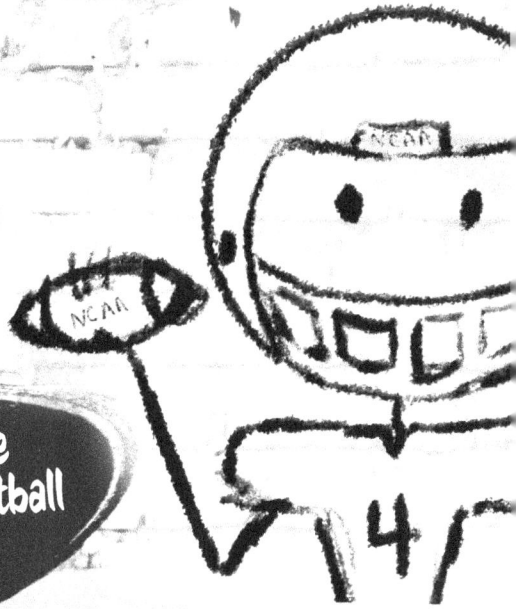

What happened this week to make you most proud of your journal partner?

Y BEING YOURSELF,
OU PUT SOMETHING
NTO THE WORLD THAT
WASN'T THERE BEFORE.

How would you describe your journal partner's attitude last week?

Why was it a great week?

What is the best thing that happened this week? How could this week have been better?

Who inspired me this week Why?

Everyone told him it would be hard to reach his goal.

How did I make a difference this week?

Add your own graffiti here,

What would you like to see
your partner focus on next week?

Why was it a
great week?

They told him
most players
don't even make
it anywhere
close to that
level.

SAY "YES"
TO NEW
ADVENTURES.

How would you
describe your
journal partner's
attitude last week?

What happened this week
to make you most proud
of your journal partner?

How did I make a
difference this week?

Who inspired
me this week?
Why?

Add your own graffiti here,

What is the best thing that happe
this week? How could this week
have been better?

GIVE THANKS FOR A LITTLE AND YOU'LL FIND A LOT.

People reminded him he wasn't from a big city. They explained how big city kids have more chances to learn from, and be seen by, big name college coaches and big name college programs.

Why was it a great week?

What would you like to see your partner focus on next week?

How would you describe your journal partner's attitude last week?

What happened this week to make you most proud of your journal partner?

Who inspired
me this week?
Why?

How did I make a
difference this week?

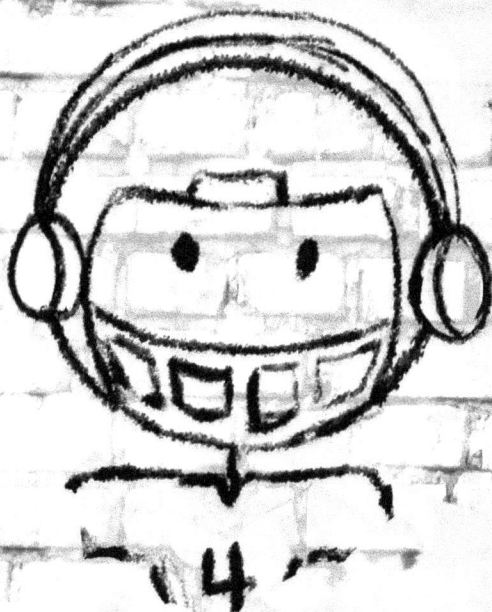

Luc's friend knew he
couldn't listen to those
people if he wanted to
be as successful as he knew
he could be.

What is the best thing
that happened this week?
How could this week
have been better?

Add your own graffiti here:

How would you describe your journal partner's attitude last week?

What happened this week to make you most proud of your journal partner?

What would you like to see your partner focus on next week?

GIVE MORE THAN YOU GET.

Why was it a great week?

Add your own graffiti here:

STRIVE
FOR PROGRESS
NOT
PERFECTION.

How did I make a
difference this week?

What is the best thing
that happened this week?
How could this week
have been better?

Who inspired
me this week?
Why?

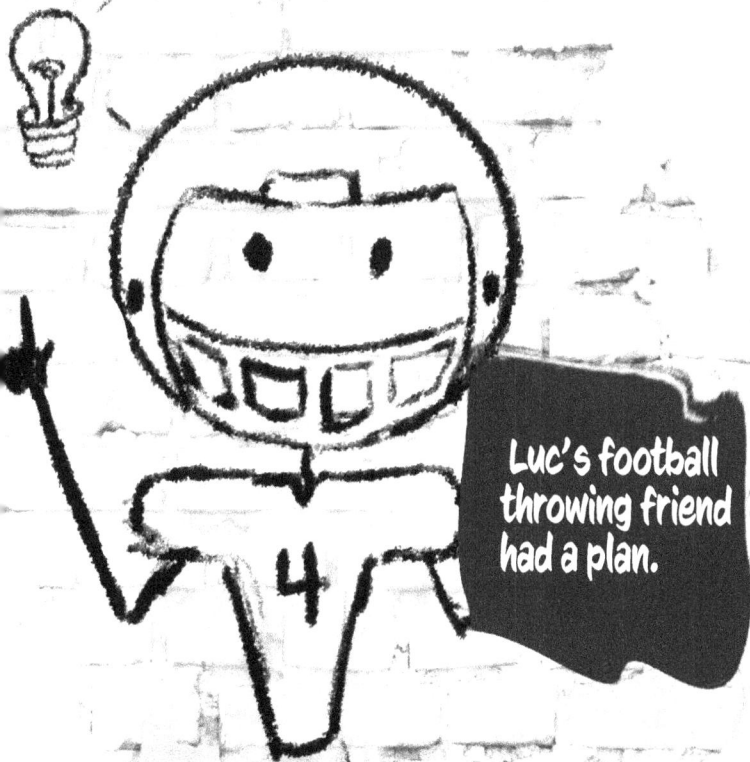

What is the best thing that happened this wee
How could this week have been better?

Add your own graffiti here:

Who inspired
me this week?
Why?

How did I make a
difference this week?

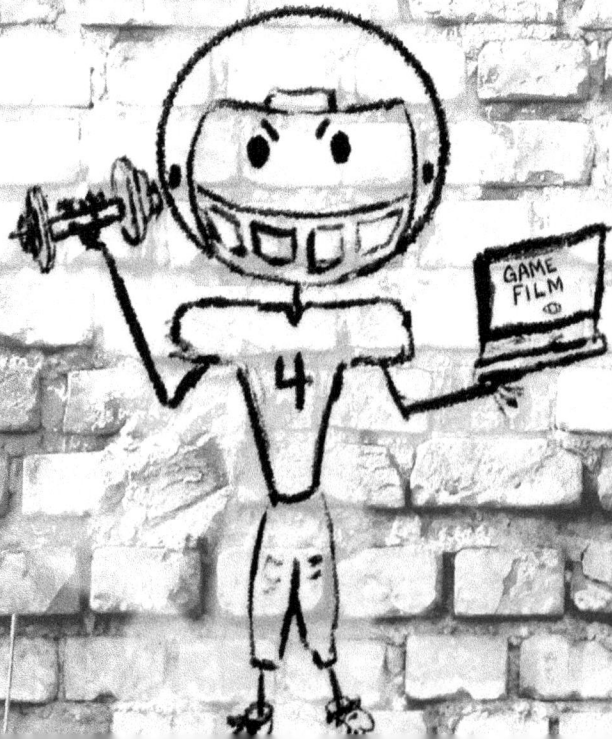

GAME
FILM

4

What happened this week to make you most proud of your journal partner?

What would you like to see your partner focus on next week?

IF THE PLAN DOESN'T WORK CHANGE THE PLAN, NEVER CHANGE THE GOAL.

His plan was to work harder than everybody else.

He decided to study game films, work out like crazy, play as much football as possible, then work out some more and watch more game film.

How would you describe your journal partner's attitude last week?

Why was it a great week?

When were you the most
proud of yourself?

All of his hard
work paid off.

In high school, Luc's
pal was named his
state's Player of
the Year!

Draw something that reminds
you of the time you were most proud:

How would you describe
your journal partner's
attitude last week?

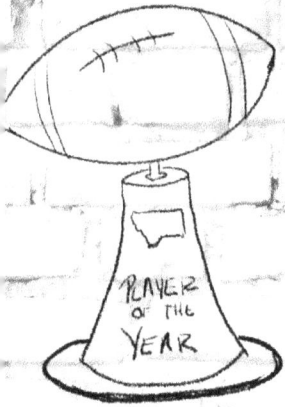

What happened this week
to make you most proud
of your journal partner?

**YOU ARE AMAZING,
NEVER FORGET IT!**

PLAYER
OF THE
YEAR

What would you like to see
your partner focus on next week?

Why was it a great week?

How did I make a
difference this week?

Who inspired
me this week?
Why?

Luc's friend
was even given
a scholarship to a
Division 1 college.
He beat the odds!

But, he wasnt done yet.
He was still on the
bench.
Remember,
Luc's friend wanted to
be a STARTING
college
quarterback.

What is the best thing that happened
this week? How could this week
have been better?

Add your own graffiti here,

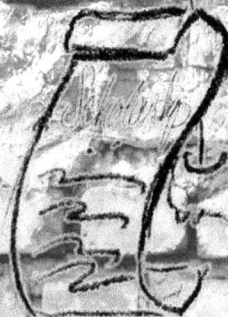

What happened this week to make you most proud of your journal partner?

How would
you describe
your journal
partner's
attitude
last week?

Why was it a great week?

What would you
like to see your partner
focus on next week?

Who inspired
me this week?
Why?

How did I make a
difference this week?

**BE HAPPY.
BE BRIGHT.
BE YOU!**

What is the best thing that happened
this week? How could this week
have been better?

Add your own graffiti here,

Once again, Luc's friend just worked
harder, studied the plays more,
and worked out more consistently
than anyone.

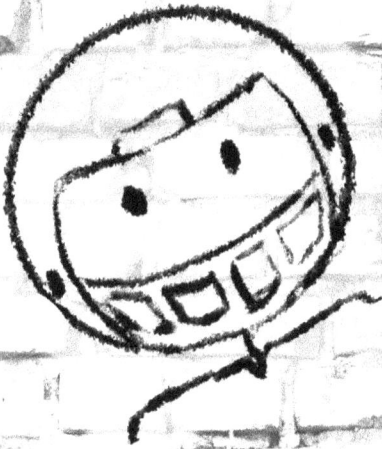

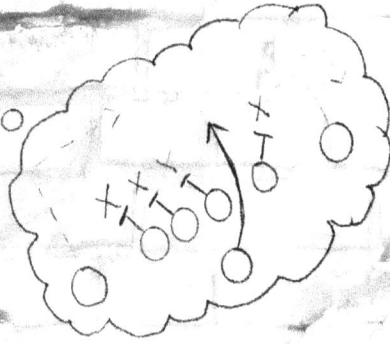

Why was it a great week?

What would you like to see your partner focus on next week?

What happened this week to make you most proud of your journal partner?

How would you describe your journal partner's attitude last week?

Add your own graffiti here:

Luc's friend reached his goal!

What is the best thing that happenedthis week? How could this week have been better?

YOU ARE SMART,
YOU ARE STRONG,
YOU CAN DO ANYTHING.

Who inspired me this week? Why?

How did I make a difference this week?

What happened this week
to make you most proud
of your journal partner?

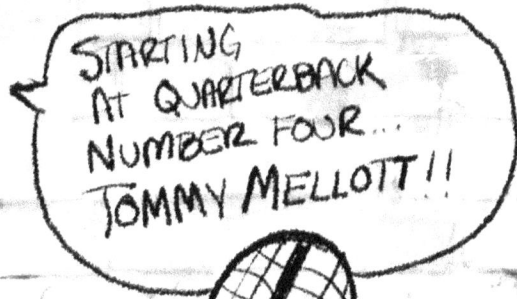

STARTING
AT QUARTERBACK
NUMBER FOUR...
TOMMY MELLOTT!!

Why was it a great week?

How would
you describe
your journal
partner's
attitude
last week?

What would you
like to see your partner
focus on next week?

What is the best thing that happened this week?
How could this week have been better?

How did I make a difference this week?

Who inspired
me this week?
Why?

LIFE DOESN'T REQUIRE THAT WE BE THE BEST,
BUT THAT WE ALWAYS TRY OUR BEST.

Add your own graffiti here:

What happened this week to make you most proud of your journal partner?

Tommy won't stop working hard, even though he reached his goal, because Tommy Mellott loves this life!

Why was it a great week?

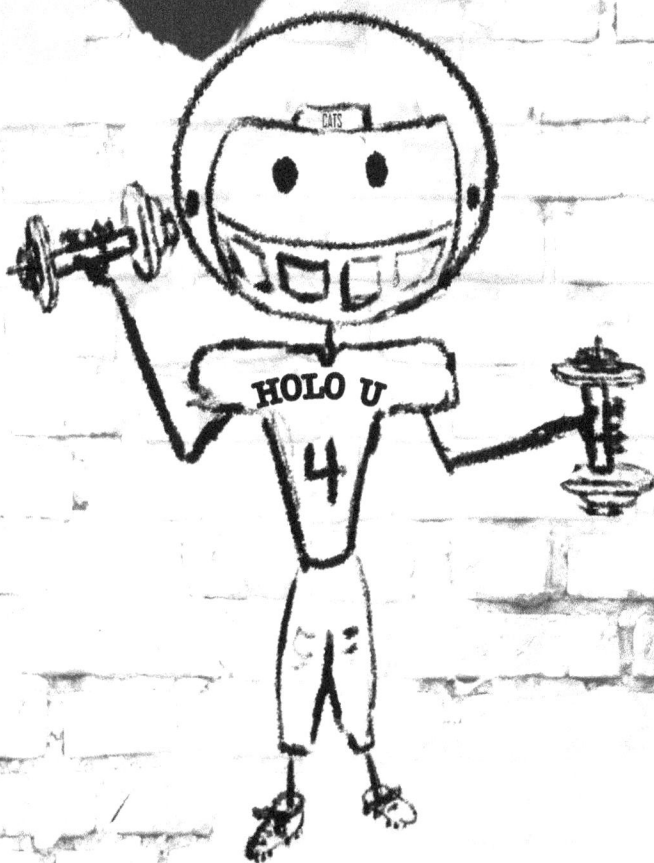

How would you describe your journal partner's attitude last week?

What would you like to see your partner focus on next week?

Who inspired
me this week?
Why?

How did I make a difference this week?

What is the best thing that happened
this week? How could this week
have been better?

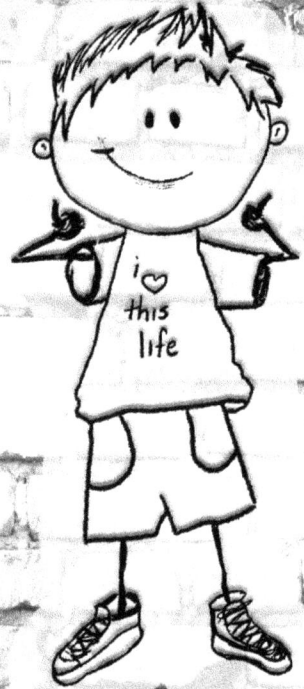

Add your
own graffiti
here.

Why was it a great week?

Real Luc has heard
lots of stories like the ones
we've told about Perrey and Tommy.
Someday he hopes to hear yours!

What happened this week to make you most
proud of your journal partner?

How would
you describe
your journal
partner's
attitude
last week?

YOU CAN'T LIVE
A POSITIVE LIFE
WITH A
NEGATIVE MIND.

What would you like to see your partner focus on next week?

How did I make a
difference this week?

RISE UP.
START FRESH.
SEE THE THE BRIGHT
OPPORTUNITIES OF EACH NEW DAY.

Who inspired
me this week?
Why?

What is the best thing that happened
this week? How could this week have
been better?

Add your own graffiti here,

What would you like to see
your partner focus on next week?

Why was it a great week?

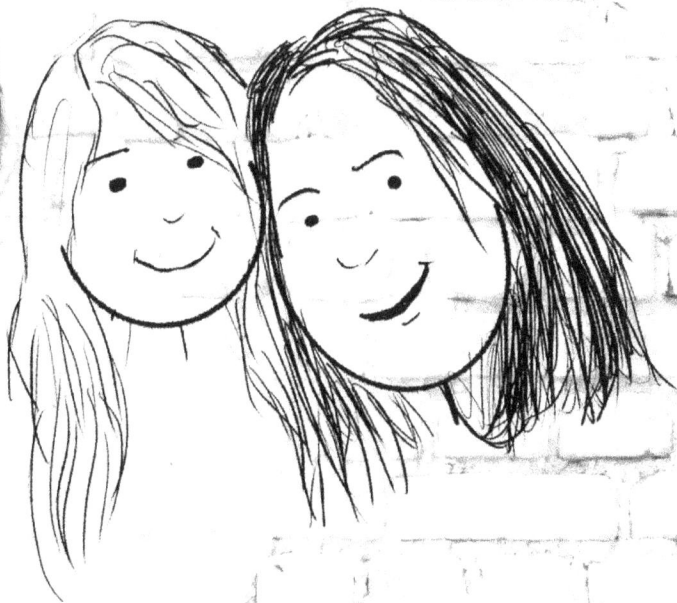

Luc has also been inspired
and helped by many people
throughout his journey.

For example, this is Tori
and Tennyson, they are
two of Luc's most powerful
influences. They are the
inspiration behind the HOLO
clothing brand.

How would you
describe your journal
partner's attitude
last week?

What happened this week to
make you most proud of your
journal partner?

What is the best thing that happened this week? How could this week have been better?

Who inspired me this week? Why?

Add your own graffiti here,

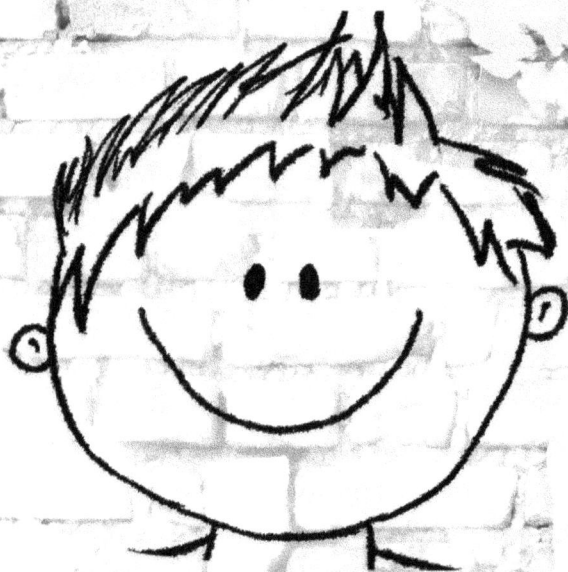

We hope you've enjoyed the journey and learned a few things.

How did I make a difference this week?

What happened this week to make you most proud of your journal partner?

What would you like to see your partner focus on next week?

BELIEVE IN YOURSELF!

Why was it a great week?

How would you describe your journal partner's attitude last week?

Mostly though,
we hope you learned
how much...

Add your own graffiti here,

YOU LOVE THIS LIFE!

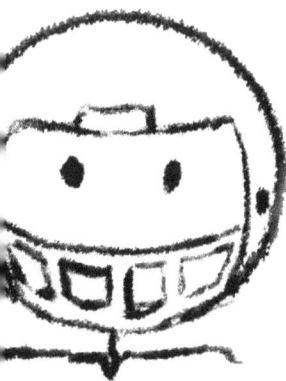

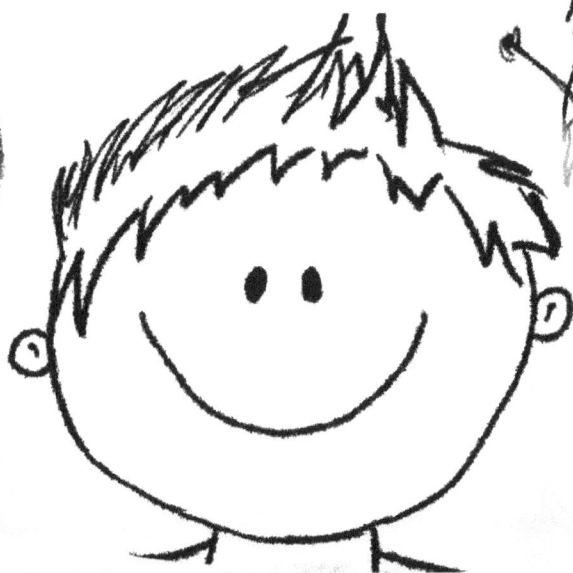

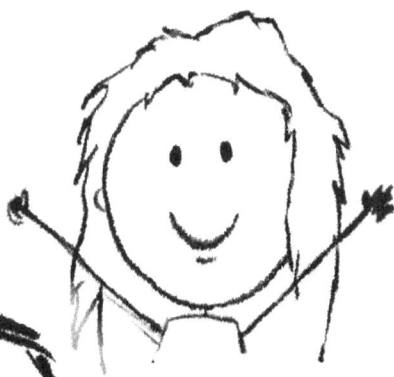

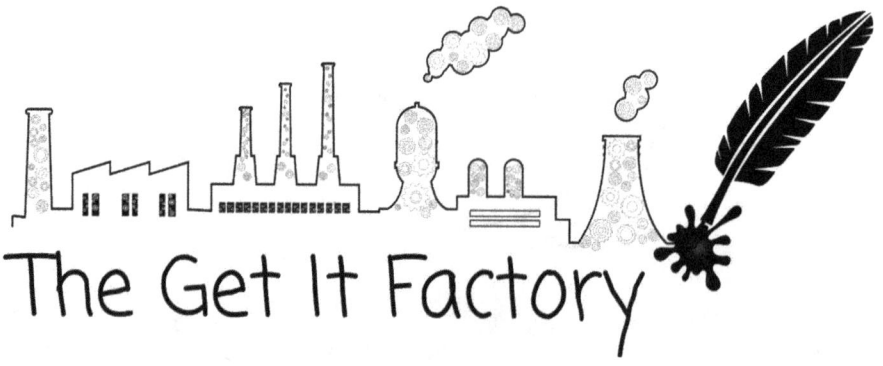
The Get It Factory

www.ingramcontent.com/pod-product-compliance
Lightning Source LLC
Chambersburg PA
CBHW080422030426
42335CB00020B/2549